Contents

Introduction

The esophagus is a tube that connects the mouth to the stomach. It is made of muscles that work to push food toward the stomach in rhythmic waves. Once in the stomach, food is prevented from refluxing (moving back into the esophagus), by a special area of circular muscle located at the junction of the esophagus and stomach, called the lower esophageal sphincter (LES). A pressure difference across the diaphragm, the flat muscle that separates the chest from the abdomen, also tends to keep stomach contents in the stomach.

The stomach combines food, acids, and enzymes together to begin digestion. There are special protective cells that line the stomach to prevent the acid from causing inflammation. The esophagus does not have this same protection, and if stomach acid and digestive juices reflux back into the esophagus, they can cause inflammation and damage to its unprotected lining.

What Is Heartburn?

Heartburn and acid reflux

Heartburn is a burning feeling in the chest caused by stomach acid travelling up towards the throat (acid reflux). If it keeps happening, it's called gastro-oesophageal reflux disease (GORD).

Acid reflux occurs when there is acid backflow from

the stomach into the esophagus. This happens commonly but can cause complications or troublesome symptoms, such as heartburn.

One reason this happens is that the lower esophageal sphincter (LES) is weakened or damaged. Normally the LES closes to prevent food in the stomach from moving into the esophagus.

The foods you eat affect the amount of acid your stomach produces. Eating the right kinds of food is key to controlling acid reflux or gastroesophageal reflux disease (GERD), a severe, chronic form of acid reflux.

Check if you have acid reflux

The main symptoms of acid reflux are:

heartburn – a burning sensation in the middle of your chest an unpleasant sour taste in your mouth, caused by stomach acid

You may also have:

A cough or hiccups that keep coming back

A hoarse voice

bad breath

bloating and feeling sick

Your symptoms will probably be worse after eating, when lying down and when bending over.

Causes of heartburn and acid reflux

Lots of people get heartburn from time to time. There's often no obvious reason why.

Sometimes it's caused or made worse by:

certain food and drink – such as coffee, tomatoes, alcohol, chocolate and fatty or spicy foods

Being overweight

Smoking

Pregnancy

Stress and anxiety

some medicines, such as anti-inflammatory painkillers (like ibuprofen)

a hiatus hernia – when part of your stomach moves up into your chest

Foods That Fight Heartburn

You've heard about the foods that can make your heartburn worse, from coffee to chocolate to tomatoes. But what about foods that could make your heartburn better? Check out some key eats you should add to your diet.

Eat More Low-Acid Foods

When acid and other liquids in your stomach back up into your esophagus, you get heartburn. The acid that's already in your stomach isn't the only problem, though.

The natural acids in foods you eat -- like many fruits, vegetables, and drinks -- play a role, too, says Bani Roland, MD. She is a gastroenterologist and assistant professor at Johns Hopkins University. To curb heartburn, build your meals around naturally low-acid foods like:

Melons and bananas: While most fruits have a high acid content, these don't. Bananas are always handy as a snack food. All sorts of melons are good, like watermelon, cantaloupe, and honeydew.

Oatmeal: It's a great way to start your day. Oatmeal doesn't cause reflux, it's filling, and it has lots of healthy fiber.

Bread: Choose whole-grain -- it will be the first ingredient on the label -- which is made with unprocessed grains. Other healthy-sounding breads -- like wheat, whole-wheat, or 7-grain -- may be made with refined grains, which are stripped of natural fiber, vitamins, and other nutrients.

Rice and couscous: These healthy complex carbs are great if you have reflux. When choosing rice, go for brown rice, which has more fiber.

Fish: Grilled, poached, and baked fish are all good choices. Just don't fry it or use fatty sauces.

Egg whites: They're a good source of protein and are low in acid. Just skip the yolk, which is more likely to cause symptoms.

You can't tell how acidic a food is by looking at it. It's not on the nutrition label either. But you can research a food's pH, which is a score of its acid content. The lower the pH number, the higher the acid -- lemon juice has a pH of 2.0. If you aim for foods with a pH of 5 or above, you may have fewer symptoms. You can find the pH level of foods on some government sites and in low-acid diet cookbooks.

More Foods to Soothe Heartburn

Other foods and herbs have long been treatments for reflux and upset stomach.

But keep in mind that while they may provide relief for some, "they won't work for everyone," says gastroenterologist Jay Kuemmerle, MD, of Virginia Commonwealth University. You might want to try:

Fennel: This crunchy vegetable with a licorice flavor makes a great addition to salads. There's some evidence that fennel can improve your digestion.

It has a pH of 6.9, so it's low in acid, too.

Ginger: A long-standing natural treatment for upset stomach, ginger does seem to have benefits for reflux.

Parsley: That sprig of parsley on your plate isn't only for decoration. Parsley has been a traditional treatment for upset stomach for hundreds of years.

Aloe vera: This is another old treatment for GI problems that seems to help with reflux. You can buy aloe vera as a plant or as a supplement -- in capsules, juices, and other forms. It works as a thickener in recipes.Just make sure it's free of anthraquinones (primarily the compound aloin), which can be irritating to the digestive system.

Foods That May Cause Heartburn

Foods commonly known to be heartburn triggers cause the esophageal sphincter to relax and delay the digestive process, letting food sit in the stomach longer, says Gupta. The worst culprits? Foods that are high in fat, salt or spice such as:

Fried food

Fast food

Pizza

Potato chips and other processed snacks

Chili powder and pepper (white, black, cayenne)

Fatty meats such as bacon and sausage

Cheese

Other foods that can cause the same problem include:

Tomato-based sauces

Citrus fruits

Chocolate

Peppermint

Carbonated beverages

"Moderation is key since many people may not be able to or want to completely eliminate these foods," says Gupta. "But try to avoid eating problem foods late in the evening closer to bedtime, so they're not sitting in your stomach band then coming up your esophagus when you lay down at night. It's also a good idea to eat small frequent meals instead of bigger, heavier meals and avoid late-night dinners and bedtime snacks."

Foods to eat

Reflux symptomsTrusted Source may result from stomach acid touching the esophagus and causing irritation and pain. If you have too much acid, you can incorporate these specific foods into your diet to manage symptoms of acid reflux.

None of these foods will cure your condition, and your decision to try these specific foods to soothe your symptoms should be based on your own experiences with them.

Vegetables

Vegetables are naturally low in fat and sugar. Good options include green beans, broccoli, asparagus, cauliflower, leafy greens, potatoes, and cucumbers.

Ginger

Ginger has natural anti-inflammatory properties, and it's a natural treatment for heartburn and other gastrointestinal problems. You can add grated or sliced ginger root to recipes or smoothies, or drink ginger tea to ease symptoms.

Oatmeal

Oatmeal, a breakfast favorite, is a whole grain, and is an excellent source of fiber. A diet high in fiber has been linkedTrusted Source with a lower risk of acid reflux. Other fiber options include whole-grain breads and whole-grain rice.

Non-citrus fruits

Non-citrus fruits, including melons, bananas, apples, and pears, are less likely to trigger reflux symptoms than acidic fruits.

Lean meats and seafood

Lean meats, such as chicken, turkey, fish, and seafood, are

low-fat and can reduce symptoms of acid reflux. Try them grilled, broiled, baked, or poached.

Egg whites

Egg whites are a good option. Limit egg yolks, though, which are high in fat and may trigger reflux symptoms.

Healthy fats

Sources of healthy fats include avocados, walnuts, flaxseed, olive oil, sesame oil, and sunflower oil. Reduce your intake of saturated fats and trans fats and replace them with these healthier unsaturated fats.

Heartburn is a common symptom of acid reflux and GERD. You may develop a burning sensation in your stomach or chest after eating a full meal or certain foods. GERD can also cause vomiting or regurgitation as acid moves into your esophagus.

Other symptoms include:

Dry cough

Sore throat

Bloating

Burping or hiccups

Difficulty swallowing

Lump in the throat

Many people with GERD find that certain foods trigger their symptoms. No single diet can prevent all symptoms of GERD, and food triggers are different for everyone.

To identify your individual triggers, keep a food diary and track the following:

What foods you eat

What time of day you eat

What symptoms you experience

Keep the diary for at least a week. It's helpful to track

your foods for a longer period if your diet varies. You can use the diary to identify specific foods and drinks that affect your GERD.

The diet and nutrition advice here is a starting point to plan your meals. Use this guide in conjunction with your food journal and your doctor's advice. The goal is to minimize and control your symptoms.

Heartburn Home Remedies

People with heartburn commonly reach for antacids, over-the-counter medications that neutralize stomach acid. But eating certain foods may also offer relief from symptoms. Consider trying the following:

Milk

Does milk help with heartburn? "Milk is often thought to relieve heartburn," says Gupta. "But you have to keep in mind that milk comes in different varieties — whole milk with the full amount of fat, 2% fat, and skim or nonfat milk. The fat in milk can aggravate acid reflux. But nonfat milk can act as a temporary buffer between the stomach lining and acidic stomach contents and provide immediate relief of heartburn symptoms." Low-fat yogurt has the same soothing qualities along with a healthy dose of probiotics (good bacteria that enhance digestion).

Ginger

Ginger is one of the best digestive aids because of its medicinal properties. It's alkaline in nature and anti-inflammatory, which eases irritation in the digestive tract. Try sipping ginger tea when you feel heartburn coming on.

Apple cider vinegar

While there isn't enough research to prove that drinking apple cider vinegar works for acid reflux, many people swear that it helps. However, you should never drink it at full concentration because it's a strong acid that can irritate the esophagus. Instead, put a small amount in warm water and drink it with meals.

a cup of lemon water with honey

Lemon water

Lemon juice is generally considered very acidic, but a small amount of lemon juice mixed with warm water and honey has an alkalizing effect that neutralizes stomach acid. Also, honey has natural antioxidants, which protect the health of cells.

How a Doctor Can Help

If you have heartburn two or more times a week and changes to your diet or eating pattern haven't helped, consult a doctor. A gastroenterologist (a doctor who specializes in the digestive system) can perform tests to measure the acidity in your stomach and see if frequent acid reflux has damaged your esophagus.

GERD is often treatable through a combination of lifestyle changes and medication. But persistent symptoms of reflux need thorough evaluation by a gastroenterologist who can find the underlying cause and discuss available treatment options.

HEARTBURN RECIPES

Anti-reflux energizing & healing morning smoothie

INGREDIENTS

1 cup coconut water

3/4 cup berries *or fruit of your choice

1 tablespoon chia seeds *optional for extra protein

1 tablespoon aloe vera

1/2 teaspoon probiotics *get the recommended dosage according to age

1/4 teaspoon coconut oil

1/4 teaspoon grated ginger

INSTRUCTIONS

Blend everything in a high speed blender and drink right away.

Heartburn-Preventing Alkaline Shake

Ingredients

1 cup Vanilla almond milk (unsweetened)

1/2 cup Celery juice

1 Banana (sliced)

2 tbsp Almond butter

Instructions

Blend all ingredients together until smooth and enjoy!

Heartburn-Friendly Chicken Pot Pie

Ingredients

1 pound boneless, skinless chicken breasts

1/2 teaspoon salt

1 tablespoon olive oil

1 cup frozen carrots, thawed and drained

1 cup frozen peas, thawed and drained

1 (14.75-ounce) can cream-style corn

1/2 cup skim milk

1 cup biscuit mix

Instructions

Heat oven to 400F.

Cut chicken breasts into 1-inch cubes and season with salt.

Heat olive oil or vegetable oil in a skillet over medium-high heat.

Add the salted chicken breast cubes and cook for 8 minutes, stirring occasionally, or until browned.

Place chicken into a 3-quart baking dish, and add carrots, peas, and corn.

Cover and bake for 25 minutes.

In a mixing bowl combine biscuit mix and skim milk. Stir until a soft dough forms

Remove baking dish from oven and uncover.

Spoon dough onto chicken and vegetables with a tablespoon and spread evenly to cover entire surface of chicken mixture.

Bake uncovered for 10 minutes, or until the biscuits are golden brown.

Chicken, rice, & vegetable soup

INGREDIENTS

1–2 chicken breasts (11-12 oz total uncooked or 1 1/2 cups of cooked chicken)

1 cup of carrots, peeled and sliced (120 g)

1 cup of sliced celery (100 g)

1 cup of chopped asparagus (100 g)

1 cup of sliced white mushrooms (80 g)

4 cups of water

4 cups of chicken broth (or veggie broth)

cooked jasmine rice (see below for directions)

1 tbsp of olive oil

1 bay leaf

1-2 tbsp of fresh chopped parsley

1 tsp of sea salt or Himalayan salt

pepper to taste (omit if not tolerated)

Optional; fresh or dried thyme leaves and 1/8 tsp ground turmeric

INSTRUCTIONS

 Bring the water and broth to a boil in a stockpot. Then add the carrots, celery, chicken, bay leaf, and salt. Cover and simmer for 25-30 minutes (set a timer) or until chicken is cooked through.

While the soup is simmering, prepare the jasmine rice. Rinse your rice by pouring 1 cup of rice into a medium bowl. Fill the bowl with water until rice is completely covered. Stir the rice around using clean hands. Pour cloudy water out and repeat rinsing the rice a couple more times.

Add 2 cups of water to a saucepan and bring to a boil. Once boiling, add 1 cup of jasmine rice. Cover and reduce heat. Simmer for about 18 minutes-20 minutes without lifting the lid (time may vary depending on stove type).

Fluff cooked rice with a fork and set aside.

5 minutes before the timer for the soup goes off, add the asparagus to the stockpot.

Heat a skillet over medium heat, then add 1 tbsp of olive oil. Wait for the oil to heat up (1-2 minutes), then add mushrooms and a sprinkle of salt. Cook until tender (about 5 minutes), then add mushrooms to the stockpot.

Remove chicken from the stockpot and shred with a fork. Add the shredded chicken back to the soup.

Turn the heat off, remove the bay leaf from the soup, and add fresh chopped parsley, pepper, and more salt as needed. Add cooked jasmine rice to soup bowl after serving. Enjoy!

Heartburn Relief Veggie Soup

Ingredients

2 cups finely chopped celery

1 large white onion chopped

1 cup carrots chopped

2 T olive oil

7 cloves of garlic chopped

1 teas freshly grated ginger

6 cups vegetable or chicken broth

1 teas salt

1/2 teas black pepper

2 teas turmeric

1 1/2 teas fennel seeds

1/2 teas cumin

1/2 cup fresh chopped parsley

1/2 cup brown rice (I used Rice Select Jasmati Brown Rice – http://www.riceselect.com/products/jasmati-and-kasmati/ I get mine at Wegman's)

1 cup fresh spinach chopped

Instructions

Over medium-high heat in Dutch oven or pot, with the olive oil, sauté celery, onions, and carrots for 10 minutes.

Turn down to medium and add garlic and ginger and sauté for 2 more minutes.

Add broth, salt, black pepper, turmeric, fennel

seeds, cumin and chopped parsley.

Turn heat back up to medium high and simmer for 5 minutes uncovered, and then 5 more minutes covered.

Remove the lid, and add the rice, and stir and bring to a boil.

Turn heat down to medium-low, put the lid back on and simmer for 35-45 minutes (until rice is fully cooked).*

When rice is cooked, remove lid and add spinach, and cooked for a few more minutes until spinach is wilted.

Acid Reflux Smoothie

Ingredients

¾ cup cashew milk

5 fresh basil (just leaves)

¼ cup spinach

½ inch ginger root

1 banana (frozen)

½ pear

⅓ cup rolled oats

Instructions

Blend cashew milk, basil leaves, and spinach until smooth

Add remaining ingredients and blend again

Serve over ice for a refreshingly cool smoothie

Pasta with Sicilian sauce

Serves 4

Ingredients

50g/2oz sultanas

450g/1lb tomatoes, halved

25g/1oz pine nuts

50g/2oz canned anchovies, drained and halved lengthways

2 tablespoons tomato purée

675g/1lb 8oz dried penne

Instructions

• Soak the sultanas in a bowl of warm water for about 20 minutes. Drain thoroughly and set aside.

• Cook the tomatoes under a preheated grill for about 10 minutes. Leave to cool slightly, then peel off the skin and dice the flesh.

• Put the pine nits on a baking tray, and lightly toast under the grill for 2–3 minutes until golden brown. Be careful not to scorch them.

• Put the tomatoes, pine nuts and sultanas in a small saucepan and gently heat through. Add the anchovies and tomato purée, heating the sauce for a further 2–3 minutes until hot. Keep warm.

• Meanwhile, cook the pasta in a saucepan of salted boiling water for 8–10 minutes until al dente. Drain thoroughly.

• Transfer the pasta to a serving dish. Pour the hot sauce over the top and toss through gently. Serve immediately.

Blue cheese hotpot

Serves 4

Ingredients

2 carrots, sliced

1 turnip, diced

2 celery sticks, sliced

8 small leeks, quartered

25g/1oz low-fat spread

25g/1oz plain flour

450ml/3/4pt vegetable stock

1 teaspoon yeast extract

425g/15oz canned cooked haricot beans, drained

3 tablespoons chopped fresh flat-leaf parsley

450g/1lb potatoes, thinly sliced

50g/2oz blue cheese, crumbled

salt and freshly ground black pepper

Instructions

• Preheat the oven to 180°C/350°F/Gas mark 4.

• Sauté the carrots, turnip, celery and leeks in the low-fat spread in a flameproof casserole dish for 3 minutes, stirring. Stir in the flour.

• Remove from the heat and gradually blend in the stock and yeast extract. Return to the heat, bring to the boil and cook for 2 minutes, stirring. Stir in the beans and parsley, and season with salt and pepper. Arrange the potatoes in a layer over the top, overlapping them slightly.

• Cover with a lid and bake in the oven for 1 hour. Remove the lid, sprinkle with the cheese and continue cooking, uncovered, for a further 30 minutes. Serve straight from the pot.

Turkish delight ice cream

Serves 12

Ingredients

350g/12oz pink Turkish delight, cut into small pieces

5 tablespoons water

700ml/1pt 4fl oz fresh custard

300ml/10fl oz double cream

3 tablespoons rose water

Instructions

• Put the Turkish delight in a pan with 5 tablespoons water, and cook over a low heat, stirring, until the mixture has almost melted. Stir into the custard.

• Lightly whip the cream until it forms soft peaks, then fold gently into the custard. Stir in the rose water.

• Pour the mixture into a 1.2-litre/2pt loaf tin lined with

cling film, and freeze for at least 4 hours.

Almond friands

Serves 5

Ingredients

150g/5oz butter

75g/3oz flaked almonds

50g/2oz plain flour

175g/6oz icing sugar, plus extra, to dust

5 egg whites

Instructions

• Preheat the oven to 210°C/425°F/Gas mark 7. Lightly grease ten 125ml/4fl oz friand tins.

• Melt the butter in a small saucepan over a medium heat, then cook for 3-4 minutes until the butter turns a deep golden colour. Strain to remove any residue. Remove from the heat and set aside to cool until just lukewarm.

• Put the flaked almonds in a blender or food processor, and chop until finely ground. Transfer to a b owl, and sift in the flour and icing sugar.

• Put the egg whites in a separate bowl, and lightly whisk with a fork until just combined.	Add	the lukewarm butter to the flour mixture along with the egg whites. Mix gently with a metal spoon until all the ingredients	are	well combined.

• Spoon some mixture into each friand tin to fill to three-quarters of the way up the side. Put the tins on a baking tray, and bake in the centre of the oven for 10 minutes. Reduce the oven temperature to 180°C/350°F/Gas mark 4, and bake for another 5 minutes. Remove and leave in the tins for 5 minutes before turning out onto a wire rack to cool completely. Dust with icing sugar before serving.

Chinese prawn salad

Serves 6

Ingredients

175g/6oz beansprouts

1 small red pepper, chopped

100g/4oz peeled and deveined cooked prawns

2 teaspoons light soy sauce

2 teaspoons white wine vinegar

1/2 teaspoon granulated sugar

2 tablespoons sesame oil

salt and freshly ground black pepper

6 large lettuce leaves

1 spring onion, chopped

Instructions

• Put the beansprouts in a bowl with the pepper and prawns.

• Mix together the remaining ingredients except the lettuce and spring onion, and pour over the prawn mixture. Toss well.

• Put a lettuce leaf in the bottom of each of six individual bowls. Spoon some prawn mixture on to each lettuce leaf, and scatter the spring onion over the top. Serve.

Tomato & spring onion salad

Serves 4

Ingredients

8 ripe tomatoes

3 spring onions, finely sliced

1 tablespoon olive oil

1 tablespoon white wine vinegar

1/2   teaspoon   granulated
sugar

salt and freshly ground black
pepper

Instructions

• Put the tomatoes in a bowl
of just-boiled water for 30
seconds. Remove with a
slotted spoon, then peel off
and discard the skin. Cut the
flesh into wedges.

• Put the tomatoes in a dish, and sprinkle with the spring onions.

• Whisk together the remaining ingredients and drizzle over the top. Leave to stand for 30 minutes before serving.

Pear & grape salad

Serves 4

Ingredients

2 teaspoons skimmed milk

225g/8oz low-fat cottage cheese, whipped

1 teaspoon granulated sugar

2 large pears, halved, peeled and cored

8 iceberg lettuce leaves

20 seedless white grapes, halved

Instructions

• Mix the milk with the cottage cheese and sugar, and blend until of a spreading consistency.

• Put the pear halves on the lettuce leaves, cut side down, and frost generously with the cottage cheese.

• Press the grapes, cut side down, into the cottage cheese.

• Chill the salad for at least 20 minutes before serving.

Baked seafood salad

Sherry chicken casserole

Serves 4

Ingredients

4 chicken fillet portions, skinned and chopped

25g/1oz butter

1 large onion, finely chopped

100g/4oz button mushrooms, quartered

400g/14oz canned chopped tomatoes

125ml/4fl oz sherry

2 tablespoons tomato purée

1 bouquet garni

salt and freshly ground black pepper

Instructions

- Preheat the oven to 180°C/350°F/Gas mark 4.

- Brown the chicken in the butter in a flameproof casserole dish. Remove with a slotted spoon, then add the onion and fry for 2 minutes. Add the mushrooms and cook for a further 1 minute. Return the chicken to the pan.

• Add the tomatoes. Blend the sherry with the tomato purée, and stir in. Add the bouquet garni and season with salt and pepper. Bring to the boil, then cover and cook in the oven for 11/2 hours or until the chicken is tender. Skim off any fat, and serve the casserole hot.

Tangy pork fillet

Serves 4

Ingredients

400g/14oz lean pork fillet

3 tablespoons orange marmalade

grated zest and juice of 1 orange

1 tablespoon white wine vinegar

dash of Tabasco sauce

salt and freshly ground black
pepper

For the sauce

1 tablespoon olive oil

1 small onion, chopped

1 small green pepper, seeded
and thinly sliced

1 tablespoon cornflour

150ml/5 fl oz orange juice

- Preheat a charcoal barbecue until hot. Lay a large piece of double-thickness foil in a shallow dish. Put the pork fillet in the centre of the foil, and season with salt and pepper.

- Heat the marmalade, orange zest and juice, vinegar and Tabasco in a small pan, stirring until the marmalade melts and the ingredients combine. Carefully pour the mixture over the pork, and wrap the meat in the foil, making sure that the parcel is well sealed so that the juices cannot run out.

• Place the parcel over the hot barbecue coals, and barbecue for about 25 minutes, turning the parcel occasionally.

• For the sauce, heat the oil and sweat the onion for 2–3 minutes until soft. Add the pepper and sauté for a further 3–4 minutes.

• Remove the pork from the foil and set on the barbecue rack. Pour the juices into the pan with the onion and green pepper.

• Barbecue the pork for a further 10–20 minutes, turning, until cooked through and golden on the outside.

• In a small bowl, mix the cornflour with a little of the orange juice to form a paste. Add to the sauce with the remaining orange juice, and cook, stirring, until the sauce thickens. Slice the pork, spoon the sauce over, and serve with rice and a green salad.

Redcurrant filo baskets

Serves 6

Ingredients

3 sheets filo pastry

1 tablespoon sunflower oil

175g/6oz redcurrants

250ml/9fl oz Greek-style yogurt

1 teaspoon icing sugar

• Preheat the oven to 200°C/400°F/Gas mark 6. Cut the sheets of filo pastry into 18 squares measuring 10cm/4in.

• Brush each filo square very thinly with the oil, then arrange 3 squares in each hole of a six-hole muffin tin, placing each one at a different angle so that they form star-shaped baskets. Bake for 6–8 minutes until crisp and golden. Lift the baskets out carefully. Leave to cool on a wire rack.

• Set aside a few redcurrants for decoration, and stir the rest into the Greek yogurt. Spoon the mixture into the

filo baskets. Decorate with
the reserved redcurrants,
and sprinkle with the icing
sugar to serve.

Frozen egg nog

Serves 4

Ingredients

2 egg yolks

3 tablespoons caster sugar

2 tablespoons dark rum

1 tablespoon brandy

300ml/10fl oz double cream

• Put the egg yolks, rum and brandy in a pan over simmering water and whisk until the mixture is thick and creamy. Remove from the heat and continue whisking until the mixture has cooled slightly. Transfer to a freezerproof container.

• Whip the cream until it stands in soft peaks, then fold carefully into the egg mixture.

• Freeze for a minimum of 4 hours before serving.

Lemon mustard vinaigrette

makes 150ml/5fl oz

ingredients

1 teaspoon Dijon mustard

3 tablespoons fresh lemon juice

125ml/4fl oz extra virgin olive oil

salt and freshly ground black pepper

Instructions

• In a small bowl, whisk the mustard and lemon juice together.

• Whisking constantly, slowly drizzle in the olive oil until everything is combined and an emulsion forms. Season with salt and pepper, and let stand for 30 minutes.

• Use straight away, or store in a glass jar with a tight-fitting lid in the refrigerator for up to a week. Shake well before use.

Variations

• Add finely chopped fresh herbs such as parsley, basil, marjoram and mint.

• Sprinkle in some rinsed and drained capers, or some finely sliced gherkins or diced shallots.

• Add 11/2 tablespoons roasting juices, with the oil drained, if using the dressing for a meat salad. Use straight away.

Beef satay

Serves 4

Ingredients

900g/2lb rump steak, cut into cubes

75ml/3fl oz black bean sauce

2 tablespoons vegetable oil

Instructions

• Soak 4 bamboo skewers for at least 30 minutes.

• Thread the steak cubes onto the skewers, and brush with the black bean sauce.

• Heat the oil in a ridged grill pan over a medium-high heat. Grill the satay for 2–3 minutes on each side, brushing with any leftover black bean sauce. Serve hot.

Moroccan lamb koftas

Serves 4

Ingredients

450g/1lb minced lamb

2 eggs, lightly beaten

200g/7oz stale coarse fresh breadcrumbs

2 onions, grated

2 tablespoons chopped fresh flat-leaf parsley

1/2 teaspoon ground cinnamon

1 teaspoon ground cumin

1/2 teaspoon chilli powder

2 teaspoons ground turmeric

1 teaspoon ground allspice

For the yogurt sauce

50ml/2fl oz Greek-style yogurt

2 teaspoons freshly squeezed lemon juice

2 tablespoons tahini paste

1 garlic clove, crushed

Instruction

- In a blender or food processor, purée all the ingredients until smooth and paste-like. Divide the lamb mixture into two portions, and mould each half around a separate metal skewer to form two long sausage shapes.

- Just before serving, grill or barbecue both of the koftas until browned and cooked through, turning from time to time while cooking.

• Combine all the ingredients for the yogurt sauce in a small bowl. Add 2 tablespoons water, mix well and serve with the hot or warm koftas.

Conclusion

No diet has been proven to prevent GERD. However, certain foods may ease symptoms in some people.

Research shows that increased fiber intake, specifically in the form of fruits and vegetables, may protect against GERD. But scientists aren't yet certain how fiber prevents GERD symptoms.

Increasing your dietary fiber is generally a good idea. In

addition to helping with GERD symptoms, fiber also reduces the risk of:

high cholesterol

uncontrolled blood sugar

hemorrhoids and other bowel problems

Talk to your doctor if you have questions about whether certain foods should be a part of your diet. Foods that help improve acid reflux for one person may be problematic for someone else.

Working with your doctor or registered dietitian can help you develop a diet to control or lessen your symptoms.

People with GERD can usually manage their symptoms with lifestyle changes and over-the-counter medications.

Talk to your doctor if lifestyle changes and medications don't improve symptoms. Your doctor can recommend prescription medications, or in extreme cases, surgery.